LET'S HANG ON TO MENTAL HEALTH

WHY WE NEED TO PREVENT MENTAL DISTRESS

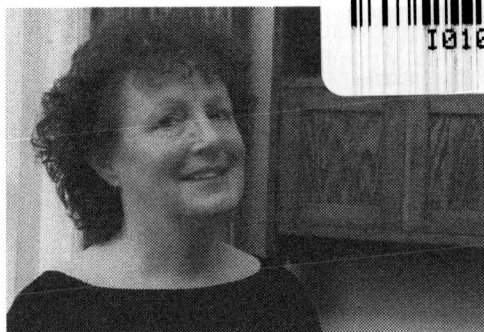

By Anne Brocklesby

Published by:
Chipmukapublishing
PO Box 6872
Brentwood
Essex
CM13 1ZT
United Kingdom

http://www.chipmunkapublishing.com

Proof-read by Ben Vickers

Copyright © 2006 Anne Brocklesby

ISBN 978 1 84747 015 7

I have put a great deal of my own experiences into this book, which I hope will be helpful to professionals and others who do not know much about mental health problems. It can also be helpful for those who have experienced mental distress, in the same way as I have, to know that they are not alone. I would like to dedicate this book to those people in the professional and voluntary sector who work for and with people with mental health difficulties. Together, I know we can make a difference. Mental health promotion and prevention of mental distress is the way forward.

Anne Brocklesby

Introduction to Mental Health

This book is an attempt to help us all prevent the onset of mental distress. I have written it with the benefit of hindsight, because I have been through a 'nervous breakdown' and been diagnosed with having Bipolar II Disorder, a form of manic depression. I have had a horrendous seven years following my breakdown, leading me to this point in my life where I feel able to write about a preventative model, promoting mental health. I know because I have been there. There are many pointers I can raise which will help you to take action, to relieve stress and actually change your future course. You will read how to intervene in that downward spiral so that you do not end up like I did by completely 'losing my wits' as my husband described it. I am not a psychiatrist or a psychologist, just an ordinary person who never thought it would happen to me. I did train in social work, and spent over 15 years working in the charity sector, undertaking information and advice work. I used my mind, and the skills of my trade were derived from having an active positive approach to work. Imagine my further distress when I had these episodes of manic depression. I could no longer work in the same sphere I had been used to, and I lost so much confidence I became totally unable to work at all. I deteriorated into a semi-recluse, cut off from employment, existing in a very lonely life at home. If it had not been for my husband, my carer, and my two children, I am sure that I would have given up. Too often I felt completely desperate, with acute anxiety, and unable to concentrate on anything positive. I was sometimes 'locked up in the house', and often could not even think of preparing an evening meal for the family. I sat, with my thoughts, feeling lonely and isolated, and occasionally my mind tripped into suicidal thoughts. I never wanted to act on them, but I felt so useless and utterly worthless that I thought I would be better off dead – they would all get on so much better without me.

Now I am ready to write about my new found knowledge to help others. There must be some real purpose to my suffering, probably at a higher level than the individual plane, if only to use the skills I have embraced to enlighten others and focus on a preventative model. I do hope that my book will be read by psychiatrists, psychologists, social workers and other carers of people with mental health problems. But I also hope that you will read this because you can somehow identify with what I am saying, and know that you need to make some changes to deal with your life. Perhaps then you can pass the knowledge over to your friends, so that together you have the skills and the ability to support each other's mental health needs. I hope to cover topics such as helping to reduce stress, keeping yourself as fit and healthy as you can by using an action plan, dealing with problems in your life, getting help when you and yours think you need it, considering the need for religion and faith in your life and getting through the worst periods of the dark night of the soul and concluding with the Government's priority by 2010 to reduce suicide by one fifth – rather I would like to call the section preventing suicide.

To begin with I will give you a brief resume of my own mental health as I now see it. To all intents and purposes I was a perfectly healthy and capable human being. I managed to cope with marriage, bringing up my two children, part-time work and at one stage I even ran my own business in secretarial services for six years. I have written one version of 'my story' in 'Move Over Manic Depression – Here I Am'. Here I describe my long, unrecognised grieving for my mother who died when I was 21, after a long history of heart trouble. It suddenly all came out when I took to writing about my manic depression – the story of my mother's early death became the all-important factor. Yet I thought I was coping at the time. After the birth of my second baby I suffered from post-natal depression, now more widely recognised as a pre-cursor to later mental health difficulties. One of the main factors considered important in predicting problems after the birth of a baby is the absence of the mother's own mother. I did not know this at the time. No one ever asked me any questions about my mother when I was in hospital on bed rest before my first baby was born. Yes I was cared for by the medical profession in pregnancy, but no one really found out about 'me'. How could I know that I would suffer distress after the birth of my second baby, and feel unable to cope? It took me some four months to feel better after the earlier nightmares, depression and feelings of inadequacy. I did not receive any medical treatment for post natal depression, so I just got on with it.

After two weeks being cared for by my family, I was then into coping at home on my own. My husband took our little son who was nearly three;

they went together along to the nursery he attended when I was working. I did not have the energy or drive to cope with him at all. My new baby seemed so small in comparison to my boisterous son. I just could not manage the demands of my life. Luckily, my husband and son got on very well, and they often did bath-time for my daughter. I took on the services of another young mother who cleaned the house for me, whilst I rested most of the day. I returned to work when my daughter was 7 months old, and she went to nursery with my son. In retrospect I should never have returned to work after her birth, I just was not fit for work. I soon developed anxiety and started to worry about balancing the needs of my family and work. My own needs were totally out of the picture. How wrong that was. After about 6 months I gave up full time work as it was too much for me, and nobody had brought up the possibility of part time work at all. So I became a full time mother and lost the support network of work. This led to further difficulties of isolation for me – I did not know other mothers, so I had to make the effort to get to know the parents at my son's school. This new life was very difficult for me, and I had no nearby support network, except for my sister, who was going through the same kind of process as me with her own two young children.

My husband says he thinks my post natal depression did not go away. He feels now that I was just becoming more and more angry as I felt the pressure of coping as a mother. He took the brunt of it. And he coped. As for me, I became a real control freak, organised as anything so that I could cope with all the demands made upon me. I was a perfectionist and never allowed myself to make mistakes. What applied to me also applied to others – they all got a hard time, as I laid down the standards. Worst of all though was my anxiety and worry. At the time I just did not recognise it for what it was. I just felt stressed, but felt that I should be coping. My husband ran his own business and worked long hours, so I set up a life with my two children where we did our best together. Life was very difficult. In retrospect now I would do things differently. At the time I did some part time work, and then when both the children had started school, I started my own home-based secretarial services. I earned good money and worked hard during the day when the two children were at school, and then again in the evenings when they went to bed. My business continued for 6 years, and eventually I brought it to an end when we had to move house due to financial worries over my husband's struggling business. All this time I just managed my life, only seeing the doctor about gynaecological problems and nothing else. I never thought of going to the doctor about my worries, and in fact at the time, I did not recognise them for what they were. There is simply no encouragement to go and ask for help – what help is there anyway? – You just have to get on with your life.

About a year after we moved, the financial pressures were increasing, my step-mother had just died and my teenage son was suffering from bad headaches and stress with his exams. One weekend I just flipped and that was it. The whole week before I had been getting up in the night and doing things in the study that I thought could not wait. When I look back I realise that I had not been sleeping well for many years. But I had not thought to go to the doctor about it, and besides what else could I do? My own needs were not high on any agenda, as I had two children and an over-worked husband to care for. My breakdown just hit me; I thought my husband was going mad, when in fact it was me. The doctor prescribed me some Valium and then the process was set up to see a psychiatrist. My sister came to help us, and together with my husband and children they 'managed' my illness that weekend. Then I started on anti-psychotic medication and anti-depressants. Now some 7 years later, after many changes, ups and downs and different treatments

I am still on drug treatment. However, I have now just been discharged from the psychiatrist, as my condition is stable, and I am now able to cope with it myself with the help of my family.

In hindsight there are many ways I could have changed my course from the nervous breakdown, but there is always the extra situational stress which turns up to haunt us, like bereavement and financial and health worries. But we can learn to cope with these too. We can make time for ourselves and seek out counselling. It is a question of developing a viable lifestyle and learning how to cope with stress. We have to learn to consider our own needs and not just cope with others. We need to be able to ask for help when we need it, or our partner or friend may think we need help. We need to be able to seek medical help as a preventative measure rather than just when the problem has occurred. We need to stop and think and actually evaluate our life and pressures. This is especially important when we have many external pressures building upon us. Loss and bereavement is one of the most devastating causes of stress. Unemployment often leads to depression. How many factors do we need before we crack? It is time to take stock, and assess your life before your mental health suffers. If it is already suffering, there are still ways to improve your life. Take stock and find out where you are. It is never too late to learn. Professionals need to consider their approach to people who are in need – are they welcoming and non-judgmental. However, do they really work to reduce the stigma associated with mental health problems?

I'm sure that low-grade mental health problems affect most of us at some point in our lives. They say now don't they that 1:4 people will experience mental health difficulty at some point in their life. I read a fairly old study by one of the government health departments that talked about the 'iceberg of depression', referring to the hidden mental health problems out there. Either the individual does not know they have problems or they are too worried to consult a GP and a psychiatrist about them, or sometimes the medical profession completely misses the mental distress someone is in. Whatever the reason, there is a great deal of undiagnosed mental ill health, and we need to address this issue. How can we learn to recognise the warning signs? How can we be proactive instead of reactive, and encourage others to actually seek out help? What help is out there? For example, when I became acutely ill that awful weekend, my husband had to take charge and contact the services of the GP for me. I was in no state to do anything and in any case I was not really aware of all my problems at that stage – I was passed it. Are there good community services that we can rely on for help when we need it? I am talking about the serious end of mental distress too, when someone is feeling isolated and suicidal, and obviously needs urgent help and care. What sort of care exists for someone in this position?

It is so easy to drift into suicidal feelings from depression. There has been a lot of publicity also about the effect of certain SSRI, modern anti-depressant medications like Seroxat, actually leading to suicide. I do feel that a great deal of mental health treatment is rather by luck than actual design for treating a condition. It seems too easy for a GP to prescribe an anti-depressant when a patient presents worries and anxieties. There has been a great increase in the number of prescriptions drafted by the GP as the first port of call. I wonder when is it deemed necessary for a patient to be referred on to the specialist psychiatrist when he/she presents, rather than to remain and be treated by the GP. I expect this depends to some extent on the services in the area, and the relationship between the GPs in practice with the consultant mental health team. I suppose I was lucky, in my case there is an active mental health trust and the procedure ensured that I was soon passed on to see the psychiatrist with my carer, my husband. I felt in good hands because I was being seen by a specialist. At that time of my breakdown, I did not have any kind of logical feelings at all, but I was definitely not suicidal. However, I was prescribed both an anti-psychotic and an anti-depressant. It was only years later after long-term treatment on anti-depressants that I began to feel as though it was all getting out of control and experiencing suicidal thoughts. I just felt so useless and worthless, and that the world would be better off without me – I was just a burden. In fact I never actively followed on from these suicidal thoughts, probably because they were not severe enough, but most likely because of two other factors. One was that I had a family who I knew loved me very much – I would not do anything because of them. Also, because of my religious beliefs – murder and suicide are wrong. Yes I needed help, so I talked things over with the mental health worker, who asked me if I felt there was anything I would do about it. I could reassure him no. But I could not change those feelings – I still felt useless. There are so many people who must be feeling pretty desperate, who do not get the chance to talk things over with a mental health worker, or whose feelings take them on that roller coaster ride that they cannot control. Some people will have been started on anti-depressants, yet still the outcome is suicide or attempts at such. I think we need to wake up when it comes to the issue of suicidal thoughts. I know the Government wants to reduce the number of suicides by 2010 by one fifth, but it is no measure of the mental health of the nation, just to reduce suicides accordingly. We need to provide active mental health services which are meeting the needs of those people who are suffering mental distress. We need to be aware that many mental health patients experience suicidal thoughts, and that the treatment of mental ill-health has to encompass ways of actively working with these feelings. Also, we need to be aware of all those people hidden away in the community who may be experiencing feelings of worthlessness and even suicide. Some will seek out help for example through the Samaritans and others will turn maybe to family and friends, but there are others who remain hidden and isolated.

The Samaritans have introduced an emotional health policy, and is greatly admired for its difficult work over the years with callers who want to talk about their feelings. They advertise that they offer a service for those who are desperate and who feel suicidal and that they will spend the necessary time to help those contemplating or having initiated self-harm or suicide attempts. Anyone can phone them and you do not have to give your name and address – they are there on the other end of the phone for you. Some of the mental health trusts also operate crisis lines for out of hours services and the new NHS Direct service is also a telephone number to contact. A voice on the other end of the phone may be all that is required at a time of crisis, to get you through that difficulty until you get your way through to the morning of the next day. However, if you need more help, it is wise to go and see your GP who could refer you through to one of the talking therapies or counselling services which operate in the area. It is wise to take responsibility for yourself and your feelings and seek out advice or therapy. Forget the thoughts of stigma and the fear of using the services because of a fear of showing yourself up as not coping. The Samaritans and the Crisis Lines are for emergency situations which may happen to any of us. But we need to find a way forward, and that is to ask for services to be widely available and accessible. The local primary care trust is responsible for the promotion of mental health services in your area, so it is useful to ask them what kind of services they provide. By corresponding with them you are helping to open up their response to their cries for help. Does development of mental health services feature in the health improvement plans? It is good to talk about your feelings and experiences and to be open about mental health needs. In this way, we will gradually help provide for the full range of services which are necessary when we have mental health problems.

I started writing this book in early 2004, the first chapters were written then. When I knew that Chipmunka would publish it for me I added the final chapter, this was written in July 2005.

The Idea of Mental Health Promotion

In 1999 The Department of Health produced the National Service Framework for Mental Health. Standard One is Mental Health Promotion. The Aim is 'to ensure the Health and Social Services promote mental health and reduce the discrimination and social exclusion associated with mental health problems'. Since then, you have often seen professionally advertised jobs which are purporting to deal with discrimination in the mental health field, and a preponderance of mental health workers whose job is to include those with mental health problems. Mental health trusts seem to have moved into the limelight and again their services of crisis lines for out of hours services have taken off. Still, those of us who have mental health difficulties have to live with our mental health problems in the community. There is still the NIMBY ethos for proposed development of services for people with mental health problems. This involves a great deal of misunderstanding and even a complete lack of understanding about people who have experienced mental health difficulties and are back living in the community after spending time in hospital. There is also the rather hidden problem of people who have mental illness in prison. Too often these inmates are too ill to take advantage of the rehabilitation offered by the prison services. They exist and pass the time of their sentence locked up in prison, rather than being treated appropriately for their mental illness. This does not equip them for returning to the community on release from prison once the services of the Probation Department come into play. It all seems like a vicious circle. All I know is that it was bad enough and difficult enough for me to learn to cope with having a mental health problem, as a beneficiary of the services in the community and with having the loving support of a family. I would say that our society has got a long way to go before it can truly call itself a caring and supportive society for those with mental health problems.

Anyway, this Standard One puts the emphasis on mental health promotion. This is a good thing. The Sainsbury Centre for Mental Health and the mental health charity *Mentality* have produced the briefing paper: (Briefing 24) Mental Health Promotion. Here it is argued that mental health promotion has a wide range of health and social benefits – e.g. 'improved physical health, increased emotional resilience, greater social inclusion and participation, and higher productivity. It can also contribute to health improvement for people living with mental health problems and to challenge discrimination and increase understanding of mental health issues.' I would endorse these views. We are just at the beginning of this process – there is such a long way to go. It is good to see that 'the framework' for mental health promotion is there, so we just need to build on it, around it, and develop extensions of the idea. I would recommend that you read this briefing paper so I will not summarise it here. However, I will refer to the research by Hosman et al 1994, which is referenced in the paper. Hosman's research indicates that the most effective mental health promotion programmes are those which:

- Address a combination of risk and protective factors;
- Involve social networks e.g. family, community, spiritual leaders;
- Intervene at a range of different times, e.g. post natal, pre-school;
- Use a combination of intervention methods, e.g. enhancing social support and increasing coping skills;
- Are delivered at different levels, e.g. national, regional and local.'

It goes on to state that the 'principles that are considered to underpin effective interventions include:

- Non-stigmatising provision – often open access;
- Needs-led programmes – based on mapping, current provision and priorities;
- Effective methods of consultation with local communities and ownership;
- Engagement with users – in the broadest sense, i.e. potentially the whole community;
- Delivery in partnership – pan sector approach to provision;
- Utilising appropriate approaches – e.g. peer led (age-specific), culturally relevant.'

The paper talks about 'the case for investing in mental health promotion' and points out that it is often made 'on the basis of whether it can, or cannot, prevent mental health problems'. Key principles of effective practice, according to the

Department of Health 2001 b), include programmes that aim to:

- 'Reduce anxiety
- Enhance control
- Facilitate participation
- Promote social inclusion'.

It is worth looking up more information on the internet about these two organisations, who do have a wealth of information. The charity *Mentality* says it is the first national charity dedicated solely to promoting mental health, offering a wide range of services designed to help organisations to promote mental health, including training, developing local strategies, promoting mental health in the workplace or advising on effective implementation. *Mentality* has a website at http://www.mentality.org.uk. The Sainsbury Centre for Mental Health is on http://www.scmh.org.uk.

The Samaritans have produced a new Emotional Health Promotion Strategy (spring 2004) which they hope will help in 'Changing Our World' and 'to benefit society by improving people's emotional health and hence providing a greater sense of well-being'. They define emotional health as; 'the part of our overall health concerned with the way we think and feel. ... Emotional health is about our ability to acknowledge and respect our own emotions as well as those of others.' They point out that emotional health is on a sliding scale and the aim of their work is to try and reach people before they find themselves at the point of crisis. To this end they wish to develop their work in settings including schools, workplaces, prisons, media and rural communities. They hope to develop projects which will be targeted and evaluated, perhaps by 'the development of a national emotional health audit'. The Samaritans is well known for its outstanding work with people in crisis who cannot cope. But as we all know, there are some people who seem to be able to

29

cope in any situation, no matter what befalls them, whilst others have very few coping skills – no strategy. 'Being emotionally healthy is not the same as being happy.' So a focus of their newly adopted health strategy of working with the media, is:

- 'It will aim to reduce the stigma and discrimination surrounding the whole notion of emotional health (i.e. not just distress or negative emotions).
- It will seek ways to be interactive rather than passive.
- It will not use terminology which is negative or has negative connotations, (i.e. it will use language appropriate and accessible to the target groups).
- It will go beyond information provision and attempt to influence cultural change and skill development within its audience.'

My own idea of mental health promotion is that we can reduce the stigma associated with having a mental illness, or having at some time suffered from mental health problems gradually. In so doing, more people will come forward at an earlier date for help with stress, anxiety, the fear of losing control, etc. Professionals will be geared to supporting such calls for help, and there will be community services provided. No longer will we be governed by the cost of providing services because it will be commonly and rightly accepted that prevention is better than cure, in the sense that the earlier we provide supportive health and social care services for individuals and communities, (nationally, regionally and locally) the less will be the cost for casualties of the system at a later date. It can now be shown that good mental health leads to better physical health – just think of the reduction to the need for services like coronary heart diseases. People who are mentally healthy and motivated will not sit around depressed; rather they will engage with life and be energised. They will have the necessary skills to deal with life's problems. They will end up being the majority who can help the minority who may be experiencing problems and have difficulties in coping. As time goes on, the medical profession will come to a greater understanding of what mental illness is and its causes. A broader range of treatments will be offered to those suffering and there will be more stories of mental health survival. There now exists some publishing companies which are run by survivors of mental health difficulties. We can read first hand what it is like to suffer delusions, or be in the grips of manic depression. We can read about repressed grief and consequential anxiety and an overload of pressures e.g. personal family pressures leading to a breakdown. On the whole, the present images of mental health problems are very negative. Arguably, the stereotype is one of someone existing on anti-depressants, remaining unemployed, with a poor social support network. We need more of these new publishing companies telling us stories of survival – see http://www.chipmunkapublishing.com. I see a future where mental health problems are dealt with early, where anyone experiencing anxiety is encouraged to seek out help. A future where treatments are broad ranging and inclusive, offering talking and behavioural treatments, complementary and supplementary alternative treatments to the traditional drug treatment approach of the mental health professional. Services of charities like the Samaritans will expand into the preventative role, whilst counselling and skills training will be more widely available to those suffering from depression. This is the way forward.

I am researching my local area's provision of mental health promotion work. I have found websites for the Strategic Health Authority, the local Primary Care Trust, and the particular trust which is our local mental health service provider. In that sense, I am taking an interest in what is going on locally for people with mental health problems. I have also tried to find out what they are doing about the question of stigma and stereotyping. I consulted the Royal College of Psychiatrist's website http://www.rcpsych.ac.uk to check out their attitude to reducing the stigma of mental illness. I found they had run a campaign on Changing Minds. The Department of Health on http://www.doh.gov.uk has also ran a campaign on Mind Out for Mental Health which again is about reducing stigma and discrimination. I also remember a poem I wrote in 2003 for the series of 'Poems for Mental Health'. I shall reproduce it here for you now. It is called 'Not Wanting to Be Institutionalised', but it could equally be called 'Stigma'.

Not Wanting To Be Institutionalised

'I haven't yet been admitted to hospital for mental illness, although my doctor did ask me.

I declined the offer because I did not want to be institutionalised.

I had the freedom of choice.

I did not have to think about it, I just knew.

I did not want to give up on the tenuous hold I had on my life at that time, so I knew it was best to struggle on.

Life at home was fine, because I knew what was what.

I knew my room, and the activities I could get involved in, and I liked that.

It was safe, because it was comforting and comfortable.

So I did not want to go in for observation, or for a rest. I said no.

But many of my friends have been into hospital and some have talked about their experiences.

Yes, for some it was a rest, a security, when they felt unable to cope at home, and it was the right thing to do.

For some they missed the independence of being able to go for a walk when they wanted to.

For others the hospital setting was the regularity they needed.

It gave the doctors and nurses, their carers, the time to sort out a change in medication, and see how they were coping with this alteration.

It meant that the user could be closely observed by the carers, and hopefully therefore get the care he or she needed.

There is always the danger though that the strength of the carers around you makes you feel safe in itself, so you want to stay on.

It is easy to get into a routine at the hospital, with regular meals being provided and the day to day existence of the wards and their visitors.

Perhaps, for some, there comes a point where they feel it is easier on the inside, so they want to stay.

This becomes the danger of institutionalisation, especially if there is a difficulty with medication, and stabilising the care needed.

At what point do we decide that the stigma of hospital admission is worth it, and we decide it is necessary?

Of course, there comes a point if the doctor decides that it is essential, and then we really have no choice.

It is at this point that the issue of institutionalisation does not really come into the picture at all, because we need the essential care.

So, stigma and institutionalisation are not relevant at the point of admission, it is just later, when we are getting better that it matters.

Then, that age old problem of society's definition of mental illness comes into play.

Society thinks that if you have a mental illness you are dangerous and need to be inside.

Then, once inside you are labelled with the definition of institutionalised care.

So, really, as yet we cannot win, until we decide to talk about our experiences.

We need to speak up and say that mental illness is treatable, and that mental health is the aim.

We may be institutionalised or not.

We may be able to cope with care in the community.

It's just that we do not want to be stigmatized by society. That's all.'

I wrote this poem in the aftermath of an episode of mental illness during which my psychiatrist had almost encouraged me into agreeing to hospital admission for observation. But I would not agree. It was not a question of compulsion because he respected my decision making ability. At the time all I knew was that I did not want to go into hospital – I would hang on to the mental health I had, just to stay at home. I did not want to go to the place for 'nutters' – I did not want to be institutionalised. I felt as strongly about it as my grandmother had felt about not wanting to go into 'the poor house'. She had made it quite clear that she would not entertain the idea of a care home, which to her still meant the poor house. Not that my grandmother needed care because she lived quite happily in her own home alone until she was 97, then spent the last 4 years of her life being looked after by her son and his wife. This stigma was prevalent for older people in care from before the Second World War, and in the same way, the current stigma is for people who receive care in psychiatric wards. There is often bad press stating that conditions are poor, and the drugs prescribed are the older ones, with more side effects. You just wonder sometimes whether, in practice, we are living in the same world as those who promote the image of good inpatient care for those suffering from mental health problems.

To conclude, it is important to emphasise that mental health promotion is an essential part of the whole mental health movement. We need health and social services working together in partnership with health service users in order to tackle the problem of discrimination against those with mental health problems. It continues to this day, people shout abuse at 'nutters' or 'loonies', and exclude them from the possibility of social employment. Yes, there are schemes for people with experience of mental health problems to do voluntary work, and yes, sometimes this does lead on to paid employment, once skills and confidence have been built up. Employers who take on volunteers through specialist schemes are usually mental health positive in the sense of understanding that it is important to have a good work-life balance, and a healthy attitude towards mental health. We need to extend this mental health promotional work into other workplaces, so that there are more opportunities available for people who need supportive work places to survive. There are too many individuals suffering from the effects of stress at work for us to ignore this vital area marked for improvement. We need a real community approach to a healthy workplace employment. Also, with younger people there is a great opportunity to improve the mental health environment of schools. Some are already in the healthy schools initiative and may have adopted anti-bullying policies. However, we still need to create really emotionally healthy environments for pupils, where the youngsters know that others will mind out for them too.

I feel that a strong mental health promotion policy in workplaces, schools, local authorities and central government will set the framework for individuals to be able to benefit from these community initiatives. It is no good just trying to tackle mental health as a personal issue for each individual affected, because there are so many common threads and too many holes to fall through. There is no safety net. We have learned that stress factors like bereavement, divorce, workplace bullying, etc., can be tackled on a wider basis. We need to develop greater awareness in the population of factors which can contribute towards good mental health. We are not necessarily happy with the way things are working out in life, but we need to be able to cope with negative factors. In this way, we all need to learn ways of coping under stress; we need to develop resilience and skills in dealing with difficult situations. Ultimately, it would be good if we could learn methods of making changes to our lives so that we can cope better. Forewarned is forearmed. Thus we often see mental health tips available now on the internet to help us with our individual problems, but we need to have a full scale community approach to good mental health. In this way we can break down the stigma of mental illness. By encouraging people to seek help earlier if there are problems, we can ensure that people actually value theirs and others mental health. An earlier approach to dealing with stress and emotional difficulties means that problems do not get out of hand, and ill health does not become so chronic. Services can be geared up to acute difficulties with long term support available for those who need it. Earlier intervention can mean that talking therapies could well be more beneficial. Short and fixed term therapy can produce changes in the ways people deal with their problems. The result can be life-style changes before problems become ingrained. Mental health promotion can only be beneficial. But to date we still need to find evidence of its widespread implementation. Mental health promotion can reduce mental ill health and mental illness and reduce the stigma associated with such illness too. However, we all need to be able to pick up on mental health difficulties when they present to us. We need to be able to deal with people who have mental health problems to help them cope with the difficulties in their lives. There are too many hidden problems – no one is taking the time and the trouble to really root out the difficulties.

The Hidden Problems of Mental Health

To find out what was going on in my area I have been undertaking a bit of research. I contacted the Strategic Health Authority, the local Primary Care Trust (PCT), and the local Mental Health Trust (which in my case is South West London) and St. George's Mental Health Trust. I was pretty disappointed with the responses. Not the personal ones – no, although these were somewhat limited. The authorities were obviously not used to people (such as members of the public) phoning up about mental health policies. In one case I was passed around from pillar to post, until eventually someone took the details of what I wanted and then said they would pass them from the Chief Executive's office to Marketing for action. In both other cases I spoke to someone who had lead responsibility for mental health, and therefore was able to undertake a discussion around the issue. But what I was looking for (and maybe no such thing exists because I certainly could not find it) was a statement of how to cope with mental health promotion and the services required to prevent mental distress. The Primary Care Trust are actually working on one now, and I'm sure that it is the most important document to be found in the local area, its just that it is not yet available (April 2004). The PCT inherited a policy document from the previous authority – the Area Health Authority (AHA) – and so did not want to distribute it to the public as their document. But it is interesting how long it takes for transfer of ownership of the power of one authority to another group of stakeholders. In the meantime, what happens about mental health?

I have discovered that my local PCT will be bringing out a policy on mental health. I asked if I might have a look at the draft when it is available and perhaps even make some comments on it for their consumption. After all, I am a member of the public who will either benefit or lose out by the policy. However, as the document is not ready for public consumption yet, I do not think that I will be getting a draft copy. The other problem is that there is no other document which the local trust produces that tells me about their policy. So, for this information I have to rely on the annual report produced by the SWL & St George's Mental Health Trust. Their factual report had a very interesting section entitled 'Mental Health – The Facts', I regard it as a useful resume of the known facts about mental health. So, with credit to the trust, I will quote various points made in their report. What I also liked about their work is that they referenced their sources of information; it therefore provided a useful background to the problem.

The South West London and St George's Mental Health NHS Trust provides specialist mental health services for people experiencing more serious and complex problems such as schizophrenia, manic depression or severe depression. Other people who experience difficulties in their lives can be treated by their local general practitioners. I know for a fact, the trust provides help and support to the local GP's from my personal experience of working in the sector, but also from being a patient in the system myself. For example, my psychiatrist would write follow up letters to my GP stating my condition and how I was being medically treated, and would send a CC to me too. This ensured that information was communicated to the people who had to know – my GP, me and my carer. Also, I know that if a GP was treating a patient for depression with medication and they were worried about their care or lack of improvement, then they could contact the psychiatrist for advice. Letters of referral were common and kept the circle of communication flowing. The Report quotes a national statistic that in the UK about 24 people in every 1000 are referred to specialist mental health services each year, but only about 6 of these people need to be admitted to hospital. Following on from this, it says that the trust is providing treatment and support for about 14,800 people, but only about 800 of these – 5% - are in hospital. It continues by saying that it is commonly known that people with mental health problems prefer to live in the community rather than in hospital. The report then goes on to consider various mental health topics under the headings of: What Are Serious Mental Health Problems Like? Treatment and Support, and Myths and Discrimination. Altogether, they give a picture of what it is like to be suffering from mental health problems and the extent of known mental health care. 'Serious mental health problems cause difficulties with thinking and emotions. For many people these are very frightening. But such problems usually fluctuate: only very few people are permanently ill. Some people's difficulties disappear completely. Most have periods when they are ill, but for most of the time they have few (if any) symptoms. The precise causes of serious mental health problems are not known. Abnormalities of brain chemicals are likely to be involved. Just as some people have a susceptibility to physical health problems like heart disease, some people may have a tendency to develop problems with their brain chemicals. However, social factors also play an important role: we know that traumatic events in a person's life and other social disadvantages can both precipitate mental health problems and make them worse.'

With this useful background, we appreciate that not a lot is really known about the onset of mental illness, so the following headings of treatment, support, myths and discrimination must be seen in this light. For example, the report refers to medication and psychological treatments to control symptoms, and the fact that other people need 'help to rebuild self-confidence and self-esteem', because of problems with feeling hopeless and dispirited. Reference is made to the standard way of helping people with developing skills and coping with the ordinary tasks of day-to-day living. Examples of these could be; finding and keeping suitable housing, work and education, resolving difficulties with money and benefits, sorting out problems in relationships, and generally meeting people and engaging in social and leisure activities. Of course, this seems completely simplistic to me, and vastly understates the problem. So with mental health problems, we need medication and skills training with regards to socialisation. I'm sorry to be so blunt with my criticism, but this is merely stating the obvious in terms of what treatment actually consists of in this day and age. Some people are lucky enough to be referred for therapies in their areas, and others will get a referral for Cognitive Behavioural Therapy or other treatments from a psychologist. However, the vast majority will not. Key workers often provide the support for people who do not have their own carers. These workers may provide the support for confidence building; help with benefits and housing, etc., for those who find themselves ill and without money. Of course, there is the whole Benefits and Advice Agency

Support Network in the community like that provided by CABs to help people with their benefits and housing, but they are greatly overstretched too. There are many people wandering around in the community who need help because of their mental health problems, but who are not actually on the statistics for the local mental health trusts. They are the hidden poor, who may be homeless, rootless, without the support of family or carers who would ensure they receive the services to which they are entitled. Also there are people who are undiagnosed with mental health problems, because they do not know they have these problems, or do not know they can be helped. There are also people who are missed in the system – the GPs perhaps do not recognise them, or the services do not pick them up. In the iceberg of depression – a lot of it is under the water level like an iceberg and cannot be identified.

The Report by the NHS Mental Health Trust also has a heading for Myths and Discrimination. 'A major problem facing people with mental health problems is the myths and prejudices that surround these difficulties. They are often thought to be dangerous, unintelligent, unreliable, incompetent and incapable of looking after themselves. The reality is very different. The Trust tries to counter this view by referring to (i) the various well-known people who had mental health problems, like Van Gogh and Einstein, (ii) Research by the Employer's Forum on Disability and locally by the Trust which shows that people with mental health problems, often take less time off sick than their non-disabled colleagues, (iii) over 80% of people with mental health problems who receive treatment and support from the Trust live independently in the local community and only less than 2% live in hospital, (iv) the proportion of murders committed by people with mental disorders fell from 35% in 1957 to 11.5% in 1995. I do feel it is unfortunate if not discriminatory in itself to refer to murders on this page at all. We need to move away from the fact that all people with mental health problems are dangerous. In my view it is usually very much the opposite – people are cowed, lacking in confidence and often incapable of doing very much at all. Of course there are people who are dangerous, but then we come on to the whole element of criminality and whether it is better to be mad or bad. Perhaps everyone who commits murder is bad? The whole sector of prisons and mental health is another area. It is well known that there are inmates who would be better off on a regime of mental health care, if only they had been diagnosed as having mental health problems, long before they started getting in to trouble with the law.

The Report then goes on to talk about Social Exclusion, an area that is currently receiving a lot of research. A report is due out shortly on the links between mental health problems and lack of employment. Again, I will deal with this later in my book. Now I refer again to the NHS Mental Health Trust report which states that '86% of people with longer-term mental health problems are unemployed and only 37% of employers are prepared to even consider employing people with such difficulties.' This lack of employment for various reasons is a big, big issue and one which needs to be taken seriously by the government but also by employers. It needs action right now – I am writing this in April 2004. One statistic they quote is that a survey of 778 people with mental health problems showed; 34% had been dismissed or forced to resign from jobs whilst 69% had been put off applying for jobs because of fear of unfair treatment. This is very worrying. I also thought it was useful for the Trust to quote that 25% of people in this same survey had been turned down by insurance or finance companies. This needs further elaboration. It is a problem I have also experienced – discrimination in the area of insurance is a big issue and very important to address for people with mental health problems.

The other problem alluded to is that of fear of crime, and crime itself; 47% had been abused or harassed in public, 11% physically attacked, and 26% had been forced to move home because of harassment.

The report concludes by stating that an important part of the work of mental health services involves helping to break down this discrimination to enable people to do the things they want. I support this. It needs much further emphasis and elaboration. However, I regard the last part of the paragraph as rather patronising – 'If people with serious mental health problems have the right treatment, support and opportunities, they can be assisted to manage their difficulties, live satisfying and valued lives, and contribute to the communities in which they live.' There are many people with serious mental health problems who have active lives in the community, and who carry out responsible jobs. There are many more people who have had their brushes with the mental health services in the past, and who have in time recovered sufficiently to return to work and live an active life. I myself have had times when all I could do was sit and wait for my carer to turn up to help me. Other times, I have tried to get work, but have been unable to cope with the discrimination I faced. I often felt more worried about the type of reaction I might receive than the actual problems I then encountered. But in my view, we all need a purpose to our lives – whether it is paid work or full-time care – voluntary work in the community, or self-employed status. Later I shall deal with the report by the Social Exclusion Unit on this problem – we all need to wake up to the problem of a lack of employment opportunities for people with mental health problems. This is a big hidden problem. It is suggested that we all do some sort of voluntary work to get us up and running again, unfortunately for many of us that is as far as it will ever go again.

Mental health itself is a big hidden problem. There is a great deal of emotional distress out there in the community, which we need to try and tackle. Various government schemes cover regeneration and new deals, organisations work to reduce crime and the fear of crime, but what does it mean for our communities? Crime levels are constantly in the press, and fear of crime is a big issue for many people who restrict their lifestyles to avoid trouble and trouble-spots. It is well known that large numbers of older people do not go out in the evenings (or in the dark) to avoid the danger of mugging, and will not open their doors except on chains. This is fear. It is also common knowledge that some people with mental health problems, known to their communities, are often scape-goated and called names, like 'Nutter', or are simply harassed whilst quietly trying to go about their day to day life. One such sufferer told me his story. He called the police, and in this instance they helped him by interviewing the troublemakers, who were known on the particular

57

estate. However, not everyone would be so proactive as to involve the authorities, and again, not all police forces would have responded in the same sort of involved way.

I think that there are certain groups of people who perhaps feature more commonly in this group with hidden mental health problems. These are the older people, the younger unemployed, and women isolated with children. Many organisations now represent the interests of the older people, such as pensioner action groups, and charities like Age Concern and Help the Aged. There has been widespread publicity for an organisation taking up the issue of elder abuse, where weaker-minded, older people were badly treated. They may be without close relatives to plead their case, or may find themselves isolated in a care home. When their mental health is deteriorating they need advocates to speak up for them, and other advisers and the professionals to recognise the problems they are actually having. This work needs to start at a local community level or in the older person's actual home. Just because they are older does not mean that they can be discounted. Older senile people, perhaps with dementia, are extremely vulnerable. Just think how you would want to be treated if you found yourself in this position.

A second group needing care and attention is that of the unemployed. Unemployment rates are growing world wide, as we become more industrialised with service industries. There are no longer the masses of unskilled and semi-skilled jobs which used to exist, and the result is more people, even the well educated, falling out of the employment market. The black market economy is well known, in our urban 24 hour society. A lack of stability and continual hand to mouth existence does not help individuals to establish a regular routine. People can easily fall into an irregular lifestyle, leading to the development of lax personal habits. Life can become too complicated, or too onerous, and one day, just too much. Life at least has a rhythm when you have a regular job, or for example, the habit of caring for a family with its day to day routine. Without this, life can be difficult, and mental health can deteriorate. It can be difficult to still get up out of bed in the morning after 6 months of unemployment, whilst a lack of self-esteem can lead to depression. The cycle of deprivation and poverty can develop where income is reduced. We can all cope in the short term, but the difference is where these reduced life styles continue for long months on end. A different culture of living without work develops, and people often socialise with those in the same position. Sometimes it is whole communities which suffer when e.g. a factory closes, or as happened, when the coal mines closed. Then it is up to community action and initiatives of regeneration to try and build new sources of livelihood for the workers. But what change that involves anyway to the structure of their areas, and the traditions which have existed for centuries. Old ways are treasured. We are often suspicious of new paths and changes. Yet a certain amount of change and growth can be healthy for any area and community. So long as the area and its individuals keep their identity, and develop strong, new areas of growth. Again, mental health has to be treasured. It is an asset for each one of us and for the community as a whole. Unfortunately many of the government initiatives are not directed at the real needs of communities, and degeneration rather than regeneration has set in. We need to get central government to appreciate the importance of self-esteem for individuals who have been long-term unemployed, either through mental health needs or who have subsequently developed these difficulties. The long awaited report by the Social Exclusion Unit on the needs of those who are long term unemployed with mental health difficulties should go a long way to pointing out areas for action. It is due out in late spring 2004. In the meantime the Mental Health Tsar when questioned about this need for recognised employment help for those of us with long term mental health needs, merely referred me to this forthcoming report. This surely is a hidden area of mental ill health.

The other social grouping I feel really needs extra help is centred on women who have children, and who are experiencing difficulties through isolation with their child rearing. To some extent schemes like Sure Start, which are spreading over the country, should go some way to build up strong communities, with plenty of identified needs and support available for individuals in need. Mental health trusts do now offer specialist units for women who are identified with puerperal psychosis after childbirth. In addition, I know my local unit at Springfield unit can cope with babies from 4 days old to the age of 9 months – a substantial time to provide treatment for the mother and to learn how to cope with the new baby. Of course there are other forms of support provided for women with new babies and other children by midwives, health visitors and the primary care trust teams. They give support in the community where health needs have been identified. However, I am still concerned about all the hidden needs – for example, people who have moved to a new area possibly at risk of isolation, those who do not contact their GP for help believing they should be able to cope and areas where they are short of midwives to offer support to new and existing mothers. I am afraid that mental health needs of mothers are often lost in the general picture, i.e. that of caring for the new baby or the children who take up so much of the mother's time. We need to value the input of the main family carer, usually the mother, who spends so much of her time looking after others that she may forget about her own needs or not even realise that she is suffering. She may begin to think that life is just like that – constant hard work and there is nothing anybody can do to help her. She may turn inward on herself, blaming herself for her inability to cope. She needs care and support, and without it has a most definite predisposition to developing mental health problems.

The figures for occurrence of mental health problems is I believe higher for women, probably because they are the main child and family carer. It may also be, that because of their change of lifestyle from BC (before children) to life after children, they cannot get a regular sort of day-to-day existence established. They may therefore become unsettled. Increasing need for space often leads to families moving to larger houses and house moving is known to be one of the highest stress factors. How can we help these child carers to cope? More talk about the need to make time for yourself helps and encourages us to think of our time as valuable and therefore ourselves as important. More help with child care at nurseries and before and after school hours can also help. More support for mothers in school holidays and half term times can give the mother some time to herself and time to recover from the day to day exhaustion of coping with the children. We need to encourage mothers to come forward for help when they need it, and not punish her by thinking she is inadequate or unable to cope. We need to value child care and raise its profile in society. Our job as mothers is invaluable – we are preparing the next generation of adults for their position in society. It is not an isolated task. It is one that families undertake alongside schools and communities in general. Gradually, schools are becoming more community orientated and community schemes are helping families to integrate into and be responsible for their neighbourhoods. The day of the isolated nuclear family should be behind us. But in the meantime, we need to support mothers and fathers who are responsible for our children and recognise that they may well have mental health needs which can be addressed. Time for a generation to recover is essential. Some time to oneself is important for us all. Let us address this hidden problem and support our carers of our children.

I think that the biggest hidden problem of mental health needs though, is for those people who have suffered a nervous breakdown and have received care, but are now continuing to live in the community. Before, when there were institutions, these people would be in the institutions and hidden away from the lives of the community. But at least they had been identified, although sometimes incorrectly. We hear stories of people who have lived 20 or 30 years in institutionalised care, wrongly identified with a mental health problem as opposed to some other diagnosis. Nowadays, with Care in the Community, we are all out in the community, except for those small percentage who need hospital care. We are mostly on medication, with paid key workers where necessary, who supervise our taking of medication, and we get on with our day to day lives in a similar way to other people. Sometimes though, people fall through the net of care. There are many people who go through periods of homelessness and joblessness, and who may have a really bad bout of depression, but fail to be identified as having a mental health problem and therefore receive no treatment. It is well known that more people present to the doctor with physical symptoms but not detail their worries and mental health cares. The result is that some doctors actually misdiagnose their patients and put them through unnecessary physical tests and treatments.

Another kind of example of hidden mental health problems is the woman who has a nervous breakdown and is treated, perhaps even with mental hospital admission, but many years down the line, remains out of touch with the psychiatrist and without medication and people believing that she is cured. But what happens when she suffers from stress, and starts talking about her childhood difficulties? Life gets out of perspective and she may take the wrong turn, for example, believing she would be better off divorced, despite the fact that her husband still wants the marriage to continue. I believe she could potentially have mental health needs and so focuses on the practical side of her life in order to make a difference to how she is feeling. Perhaps the thrill of a new relationship is what she is after, as an alternative to finding anything of interest in her day to day life. What about the man who says he wants to move to a new job because he is finding the current job a strain, and in between there are times he really feels he just cannot cope any longer with all the stresses and strains affecting him? Would he go along to his GP and have a consultation? Or does he bury his head in the sand and pretend that he is coping? Why do we take one course of action rather than another? It is said that we often cannot face up to the fact that we are under stress and tend to be in denial, so we do not present it to the doctor, or if we do, it is with some other physical problem. Other people may tend to blank out their emotions so that they can hide, at least to themselves, the difficulties they are experiencing. They therefore live their lives on a different kind of a plane, almost detached, which in itself is not the healthiest perspective to have.

Social Inclusion through More Mental Health Promotion

Social exclusion in itself can lead to mental distress, so that in the end the individual's difficulties stem largely from the social exclusion which resulted from earlier illness, and not the condition itself. We need to remember we want to prevent mental distress.

There are enough problems to deal with in trying to get over mental health difficulties without having to deal with the problems of social exclusion which are then thrown up at us from society. We often try to get back into work through the 'volunteer' route, but this can become a backwater. We may initially thrive, but then start to lose skills again, as we realise that although we are accepted in this volunteer role, we cannot get out further again into the wider employment market and get a paid job. So unemployment and mental health needs is a big issue, and the Social Exclusion Unit brought out a report in June 2004, where they argued that more needs to be done to reduce the stigma and discrimination in this area. In early 2005 I wrote to John Prescott, at the Office of the Deputy Prime Minister, and he replied assuring me that his office would continue to be involved in the field of mental health to improve the position of people who had experienced mental health difficulties and the resultant loss of employment. I found this very encouraging. Improving the lot of individuals can at the same time improve the economy and help reduce these 'structural barriers to mental health'. The individual's story is a political one too.

We now have the Disability Discrimination Act which also came in during 2004, and we have this big issue of whether we should tell others about our mental health condition, if it is a long term condition, or whether we should just keep quiet. If we keep quiet and an employer discovers it later then it could be grounds for dismissal. However, if we are on medication and are substantially affected by our mental ill health, then it could well be the best thing to let the employer know. Reasonable adjustments can be made, which could enable us to hold on to our jobs. The Disability Employment Adviser can help arrange special equipment or particular work conditions which may help us take on a job, or even hold on to a job. The difficulty is that if we do tell a potential employer about our mental health condition; that could be the last time we hear again from the employer. I think it is best to be upfront about mental health difficulties, even if they are in the past, and the condition is stabilised, and the more people who are open about their experiences with mental ill health, then the more acceptable the condition becomes generally. We can categorically assert that our experience as a user of mental health services gives us a special expertise and knowledge which could be very useful to an employer. For example, some NHS trusts advertise jobs which may request this expertise, or encourage applications from people with a history of mental illness to compete with others for the jobs – the best person gets the job. Disability is not the bar it once was. We need to make sure that practice does follow this new legislation.

My local mental health trust for St George's and South West London actually has a specialist 'User Employment Programme' which supports this mental health experience and offers ongoing support to workers and would be workers, who have mental health conditions. They are also front runners in providing a Work Preparation Course for unemployed people referred through the Job Centres. I have been lucky enough to have just emerged from such a course, with the benefit of a 3 week self-confidence and self esteem course, followed by a work experience placement within the Trust. I have learned a lot about the NHS, and now have recent up-to-date work experience through a highly organised and professional course. I would recommend that more of these courses are available for unemployed people with mental health difficulties, who are able to work and just need a bit of supported encouragement like I did to get back into the workforce. Such schemes can help reduce mental distress. It is so dispiriting to be looking for work, but knowing that no employer is going to take you because you are not currently working, have had a break because of a health condition and do not have references. Such courses help you get a different perspective on life, and they give you practical support to get back into work. We need that help, otherwise change just does not happen - society is too full of discrimination, and ignorance about mental health.

But we can help change society. We can speak up about our condition, and get involved in the local community. We need a helping hand from local groups, like voluntary organisations and spiritual groups. My local community has a special support group for individuals with a history of mental health difficulties, who are volunteering. I used that service for a year and a half whilst I was volunteering after bouts of illness. I was also invited along to my local church group for people who had experienced mental ill health and who needed extra support in a weekly prayer group which offered also a social occasion for tea and a bit of chat. Both of these groups have been very supportive. I do hope that these services are available in other areas too, and if not, if you are reading this, and work in the health and social care sector, then perhaps you can help to set up such groups. I hope that spiritual and faith leaders can reach out to find those of us who are isolated in spirit and living in fear of the future. Such measures to encourage inclusion and participation will reduce the feelings of despair and loneliness that many service users feel. It will also do a great job in eliminating that feeling of 'alienation' from mainstream life.

What is happening globally? The World Health Organization met in Helsinki in January 2005, for a

European Ministerial Conference on Mental Health. 'An ounce of prevention is worth a pound of cure' was the subheading to their paper, 'Mental Health Promotion and Mental Disorder Prevention'. They state, 'a lack of positive mental health is a threat to public health, the quality of life and the stability of Europe. The direct and indirect consequences of mental disorders lead to enormous health and social burdens, including discrimination and marginalisation, reduced social cohesion and negative economic effects'. They go on to say that 'a public mental health policy should include the promotion of mental health and the prevention of mental disorders, in addition to treatment and rehabilitation. Unfortunately to date, there has been little implementation of evidence-based approaches to promotion and prevention across Europe.' I agree when they say mental health is everybody's business, and that partnership working is required!!

But our Mental Health 'Tsar' Louis Appleby published his '5 Years On' report in December 2004 – that is five years on from the introduction of the National Service Framework in 1999. He too concludes that not enough has been done about mental health promotion and more investment is needed. Areas of work in mental health promotion need to be around reducing stigma and discrimination - and the report states 'changing attitudes is a long term challenge' - reducing homelessness and working with and including black and ethnic minority groups and individuals. The report makes interesting reading, once I got a hold of it, because I think it went out of print for a while. Other conclusions refer to the need to promote services for carers and to improve inpatient services.

On an individual level we can all try and do something to make others aware of mental health needs. We can all learn to be more open about our emotions and our feelings, and recognise that talking about them is good for our health. NIMHE, the National Institute for Mental Health in England (http://www.nimhe.org.uk) has various resources and articles and keeps you up to date with what is happening in the mental health field. We need to make sure that this information is widely broadcast to the general population, so there is a greater understanding of mental health needs and the most up to date knowledge is applied in the care of people who are ill. We need to hear more from people who have experienced mental distress, so that more information can be gathered on feelings of distress, of anxiety, and for example, of what it is really like to have psychosis.

I see that the NIMHE website also has some guides to coping with physical health, which is an area that is often neglected by psychiatrists and GPs, when they focus in on the mind. There are some very useful guides for both care-workers and individuals suffering from mental health problems. One of them recommends the use of an 'About Me' card which sounds an excellent idea. When I was in the grips of psychosis I needed to be reminded who I was, and a brief card which gave me my details, and who was there to support me and which groups I was involved with, would have been a useful piece of identity to hold on to. Then, this could be produced for all care workers and professionals, and visitors who need to see what is happening in this person's life. If necessary, if there are no support systems in place, then they can be introduced in an appropriate way. This could happen for people in acute care in inpatient wards, and also in the community, and especially in times of crisis when the carer may need emotional support themselves, because of the extra stress. We need to know that someone cares for us, whether it is the local church support group, or the local voluntary visitor, or the supportive nurse attached to the GP practice, or the psychologist who can offer 'talking therapies'. Imagine the desolation you might feel if you could not add anyone's name to your card.

So yes, we need to prevent mental distress.

www.ingramcontent.com/pod-product-compliance
Lightning Source LLC
Chambersburg PA
CBHW031219270326
41931CB00006B/617